A First-Time Mom's Guide to Pregnancy:

Pregnancy is a journey full of new experiences, emotions, and challenges. Whether it's your first time or your fifth, the road to motherhood is never the same for any two women. That's why this ebook is written with you in mind—offering guidance, reassurance, and support as you navigate the beautiful and sometimes messy adventure of pregnancy.

Written by Noémi Wognin, a singer, songwriter, and first-time mom who knows what it's like to feel overwhelmed and underprepared, this guide is filled with personal insights, helpful tips, and real advice you can trust. From understanding early pregnancy signs to preparing for labor and delivery, Noémi shares the knowledge she's gathered from other mamas and her own life-changing experience.

In these pages, you'll find:

- Tips for managing common pregnancy symptoms like nausea, back pain, and fatigue.
- Provide helpful advice on what you need to buy before your baby arrives.
- Simple, relatable guidance on preparing for labor and postpartum care.
- Warm and nurturing support to remind you that you are not alone!

Whether you're worried about what's to come or excited about the miracle of life growing inside you, this ebook is here to offer the reassurance and gentle humor that every first-time mom needs.

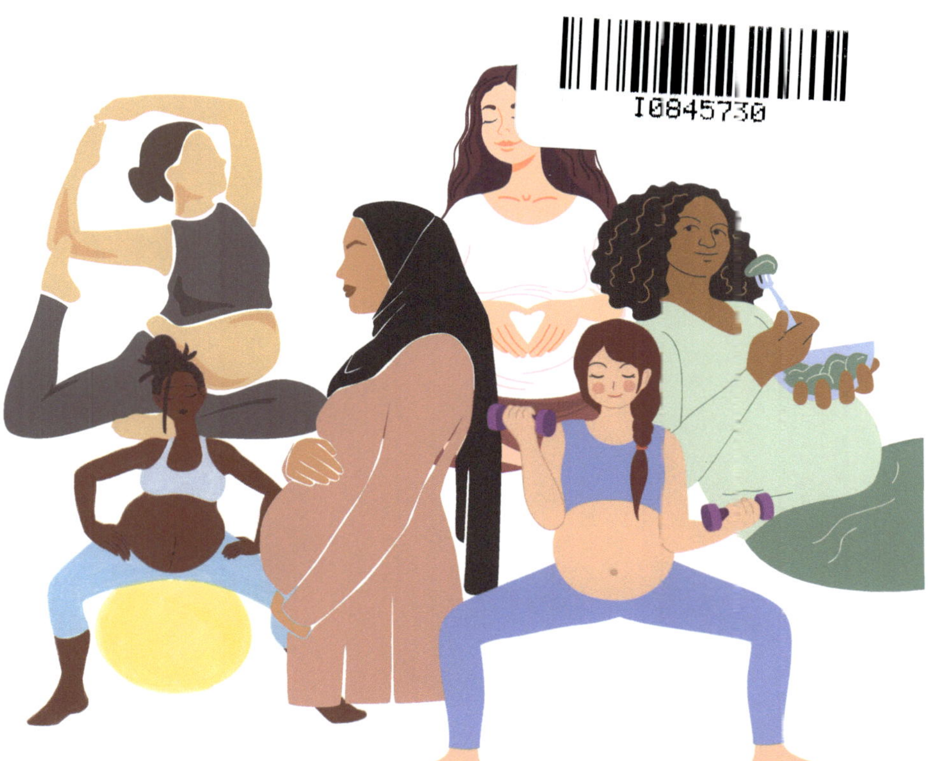

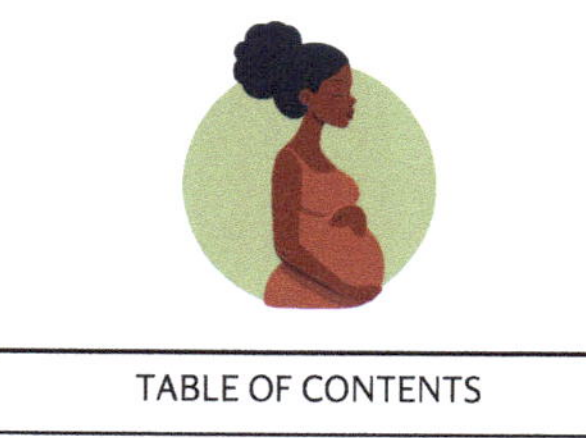

TABLE OF CONTENTS

Introduction:
Welcome to This Beautiful Journey

Dear mama-to-be,

First of all, congratulations. You're about to embark on a life-changing adventure, one that will have you questioning everything you thought you knew about yourself and loving more deeply than you ever imagined. And guess what? That's all perfectly normal. The first time you see those two pink lines on the test, the journey begins. One minute you're filled with excitement, and the next you're wondering, "Wait, what have I gotten myself into?"

This book is here to walk alongside you during the most beautiful—and sometimes challenging—time of your life.

Pregnancy and early motherhood are filled with so many "firsts," so many moments that will leave you in awe of the new little person you're about to meet, and so many moments where you might wonder if you're doing it right (spoiler: you are).

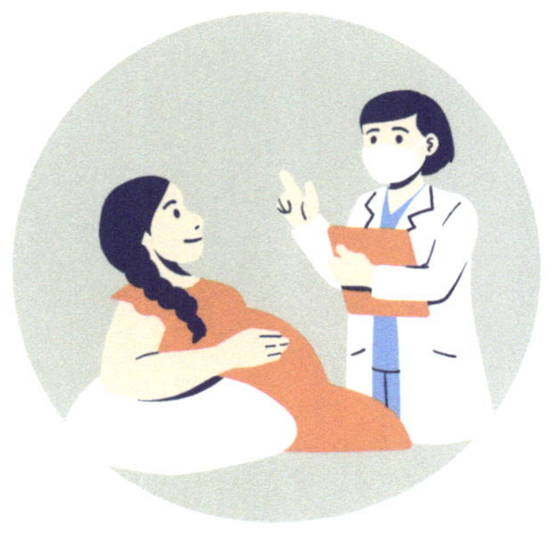

EARLY SIGNS OF PREGNANCY & THE FIRST TRIMESTER

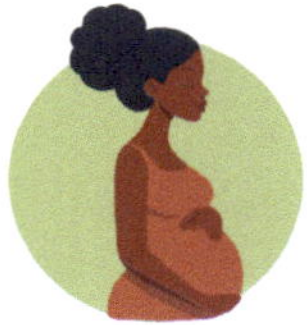

The first trimester is like a mystery novel where you're the detective, trying to figure out if the changes you're feeling are "normal" or if you've just signed up for a completely different plot twist. You may find yourself exhausted by 2 p.m., suddenly craving foods you would never touch before (pickle-and-peanut-butter sandwich, anyone?), or feeling nauseous every time you step into the kitchen.

The Early Signs: Is It Really Pregnancy, or Did I Just Have Too Much Coffee?

Some women notice pregnancy symptoms right away, while others don't feel much until later on. Here's what to watch out for in those first few weeks:

- Fatigue: You may feel like you've just run a marathon... in your sleep. Fatigue can hit early, and it's okay to take naps whenever possible. Your body is doing some serious work in these early weeks, and it's perfectly okay to slow down.
- Morning Sickness: Spoiler alert: it's not just in the morning. Morning sickness can strike at any time of the day or night. You might feel nauseous or even throw up, but remember, it's a phase, and it will pass. Try small meals, ginger tea, and staying hydrated.
- Tender Breasts: If your boobs suddenly feel like they're in the spotlight for all the wrong reasons, it's totally normal. They're preparing for the big job of feeding your baby!
- Frequent Bathroom Breaks: You'll soon realize you'll be spending more time in the bathroom than you ever thought possible. Frequent urination is common in early pregnancy because of hormonal changes and increased blood flow. It's also a good excuse to get a few extra bathroom breaks in at work.

The First Trimester: Growing and Changing

The first trimester can feel like a whirlwind of emotions and physical changes. But here's the important part: you are growing a little human! That is no small feat. While your body may feel like it's being stretched, pulled, and generally "rearranged," rest assured that these changes are all part of the process. It's your body's way of making room for your baby to grow.

It's okay to take things slow. Let your body rest, ask for help when you need it, and don't be too hard on yourself. You're doing something incredible.

One symptom that may occur during the first trimester which is surprisingly the one that made me take a pregnancy test is constipation. It is a common but not so talked about issue many women face, especially as hormonal changes, growing baby bellies, and changes in diet can all play a role in slowing down digestion. Here are some gentle, practical tips to help relieve constipation during pregnancy, along with some soothing advice:

- Stay Hydrated: Drink plenty of water—at least 8–10 glasses a day. Proper hydration softens stool and aids digestion. Start your day with a warm beverage, like lemon water or ginger tea, to stimulate digestion and provide relief.

- Intake High-Fiber Foods/ Supplements: Include whole wheat bread, fruits like mango and kiwi, vegetables, and legumes in your diet. Fiber helps bulk up stool and keep things moving.

- Add Probiotics: Foods like yogurt, kefir, or fermented vegetables like Kimchi promote healthy gut bacteria and support digestion.

- Go Easy on Iron Supplements: If possible, talk to your doctor about iron alternatives. High iron doses can sometimes worsen constipation, although they could help with fatigue.

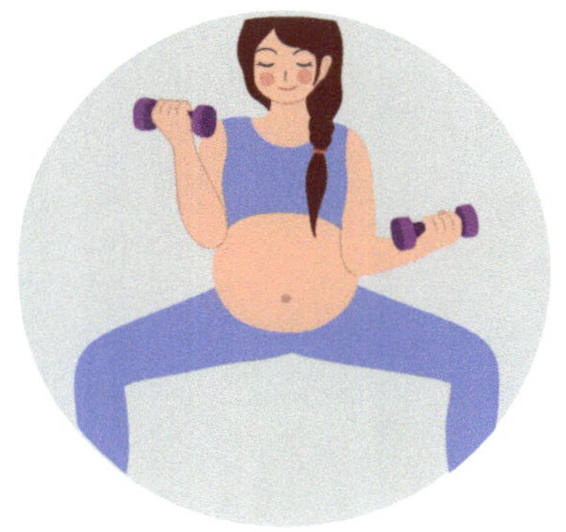

CHAPTER TWO

IS IT SAFE TO EXERCISE WHILE PREGNANT?

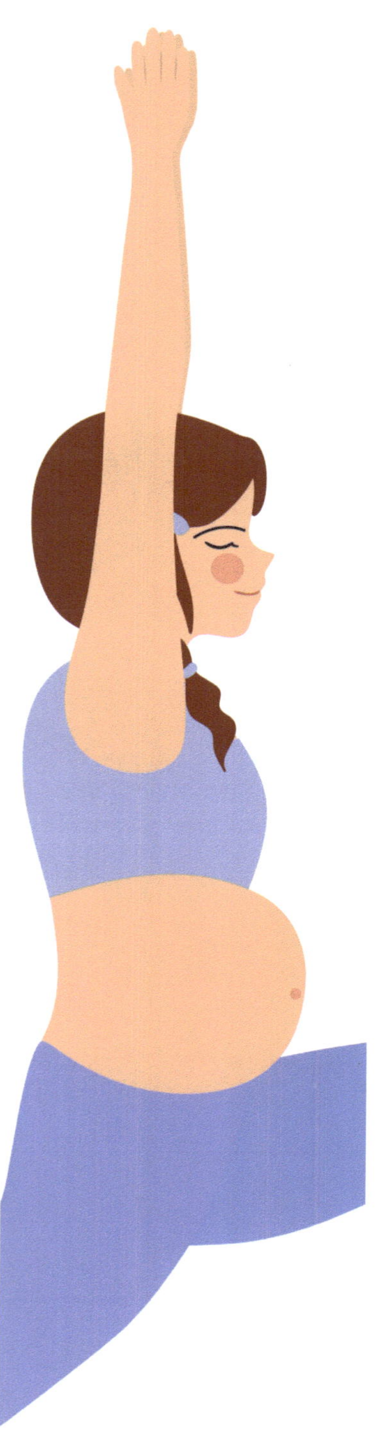

If you've been keeping up with your regular workouts, or maybe you've just discovered how great it feels to move your body, and now you're wondering: Is it safe to exercise while pregnant? The short answer: Yes, but it depends. Your body is working overtime, but that doesn't mean you have to stop being active altogether.

Pregnancy Doesn't Mean a Total Fitness Break (Unless You Want It To)

In fact, staying active during pregnancy is often encouraged (as long as your doctor gives you the green light). Low-impact activities like hiking, swimming, and prenatal yoga helped me with things like reducing stress, improving my circulation, and relieving some of those aches and pains. But if you've never been active before, now may not be the best time to start running marathons or attempting a personal best on the squat rack.

Keep It Simple and Gentle

Here's the key: listen to your body. You may find that what felt comfortable a few weeks ago isn't quite so easy now. Be kind to yourself and adjust your routine accordingly.

Tip: Exercise is a wonderful way to de-stress, but if you find yourself getting winded, dizzy, or in any sort of pain, stop and check in with your doctor. Rest is just as important as movement during pregnancy.

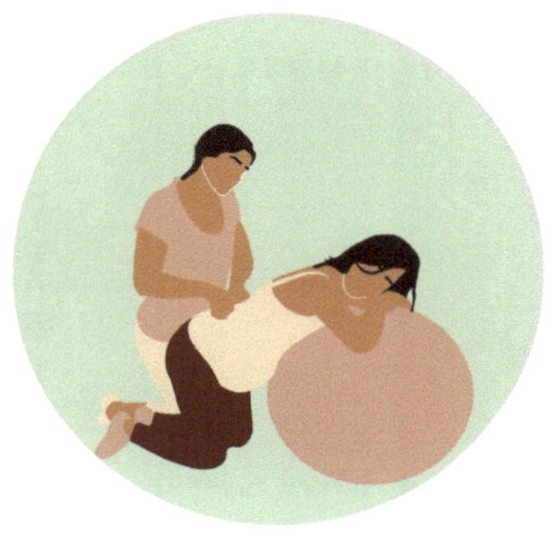

DEALING WITH PREGNANCY ACHES AND PAINS

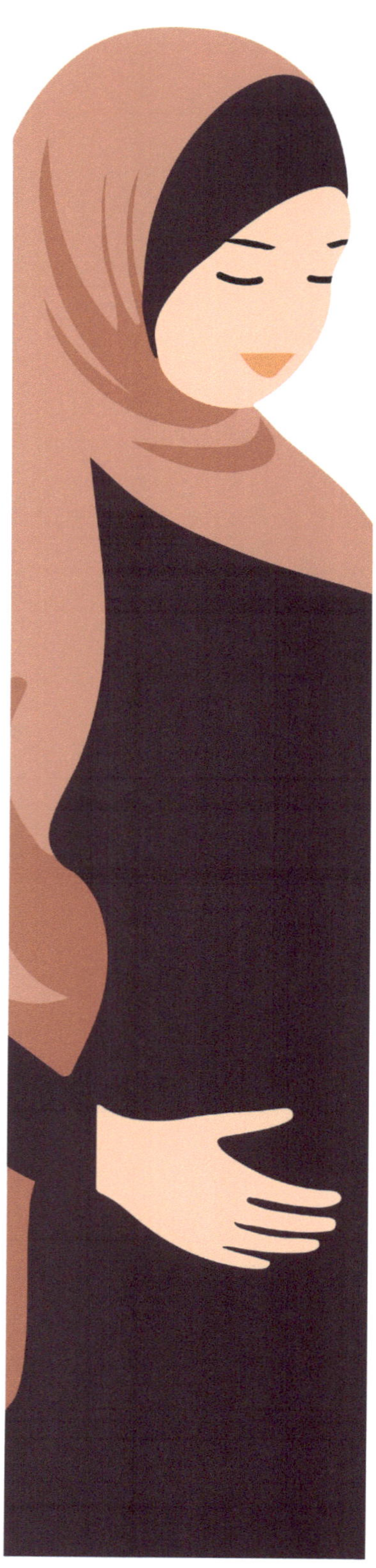

Pregnancy comes with its fair share of aches and pains, and while it's totally normal to experience discomfort, that doesn't make it any less annoying.

The Realities of Pregnancy: Aches, Pains, and Soreness

From back pain to swollen feet, pregnancy often means feeling like your body is carrying around an extra load. Here's how to deal with the common discomforts:

- Back pain: You're growing a baby, which means that your uterus is stretching to make space for baby. Your body's center of gravity is also shifting, so try wearing supportive shoes, using a body pillow when sleeping, and doing gentle stretching to help alleviate some of the strain.

- Swollen feet and ankles: Pregnancy hormones cause your body to retain extra fluid, and that can mean swollen feet. Elevating your feet when sitting, staying hydrated, and wearing comfortable shoes can help. But the ultimate advice I can provide to you is to try reducing salt intake and treat yourself with Epsom salt baths. Make sure that the water is lukewarm to avoid dizziness.

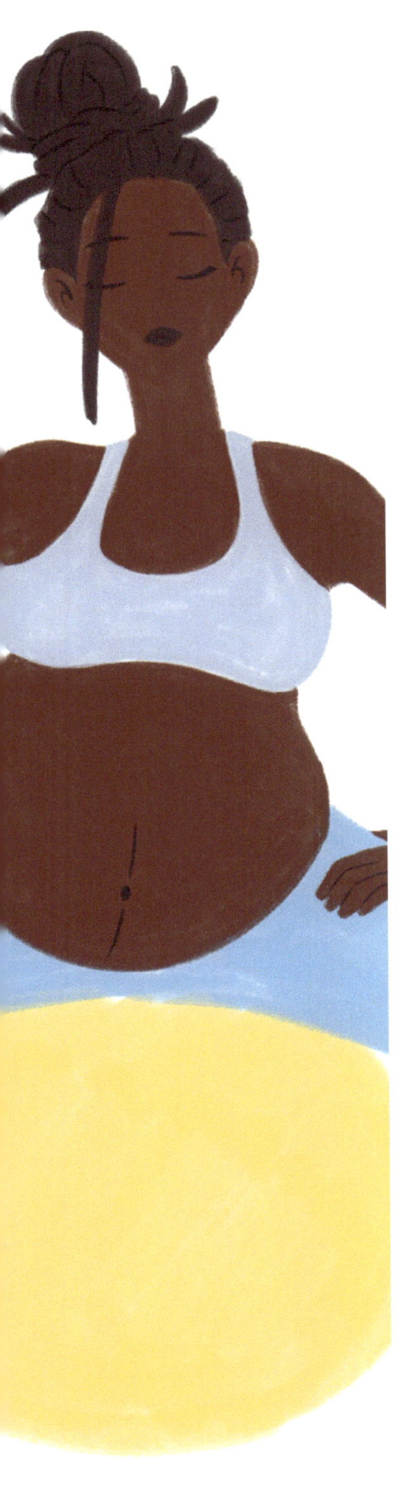

- Arm/Leg Cramps: Pregnancy cramps are no joke. Stretch your arms and legs before bed, and make sure you're getting enough magnesium in your diet.

It's All Temporary

While pregnancy aches can be frustrating, keep in mind that these discomforts are usually short-lived. And once your baby arrives, your body will begin to heal and adjust again. It's all part of the process.

Tips:
- Stretch and Strengthen: Gentle stretches like pelvic tilts, cat-cow, and hip openers can relieve tension in your lower back. Prenatal yoga or swimming can help keep your muscles strong and flexible.

- Heat or Cold Therapy: A warm compress or heating pad on your back can ease tension, while a cold pack can reduce inflammation if you're feeling swollen or sore.

- Avoid Heavy Lifting: Pregnancy puts extra strain on your back, so avoid heavy lifting. When picking things up, bend your knees, not your back.

- Prenatal Massage or Chiropractic Care: A massage from a certified prenatal therapist can help relieve tight muscles, and seeing a chiropractor who specializes in pregnancy can align your spine and reduce pain.

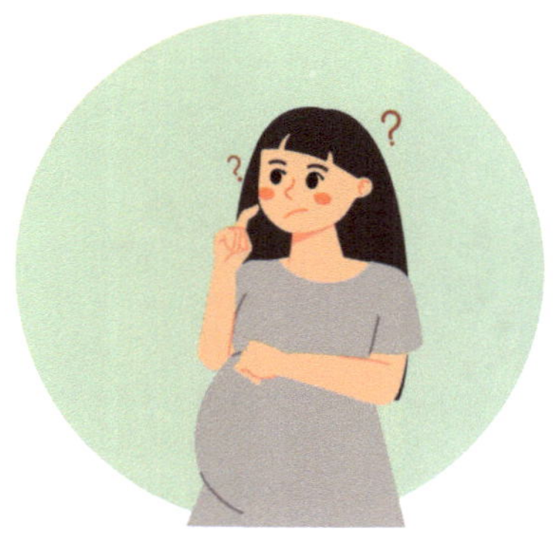

ESSENTIAL THINGS I NEED TO BUY BEFORE THE BABY ARRIVES

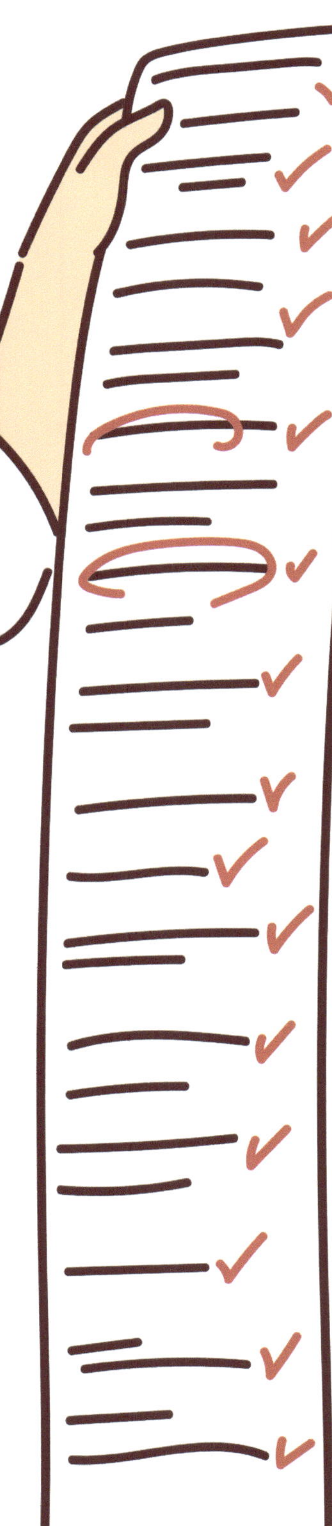

There's no shortage of baby gear out there, and the shopping lists can be overwhelming for first-time moms. Let's break it down to the essentials so you can save your energy for those precious moments with your little one.

The Essentials You Really Need (No, You Don't Need Five Cribs)

- Car Seat: You need this before you can leave the hospital. It's non-negotiable, so get it installed ahead of time.

- Clothing: You'll need a few basics like onesies, socks, and hats. But remember, babies grow fast, so don't overdo it.

- Diapers: You'll go through a lot of diapers, so stock up. Both cloth and disposable options are available—go with what feels right for you.

- Swaddle Blankets: Babies love being snug and swaddled, and these blankets are a lifesaver.

- Feeding Supplies: Whether you plan to breastfeed or bottle-feed, make sure you have a plan in place. If breastfeeding, invest in a good nursing bra and nipple cream. I do not recommend formula feeding for dietary reasons but as a new mom we do what we can and it's ok ! If formula feeding stock up on bottles and formula.

Tip: Don't stress about buying everything at once. Babies don't need half the things you'll see on Pinterest. Focus on the basics first and buy as you go.

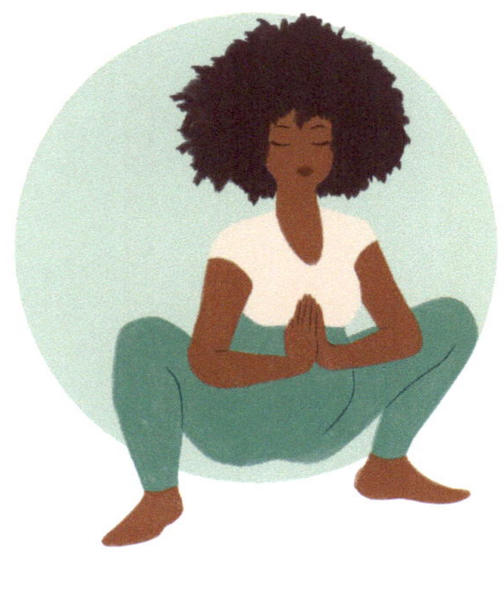

CHAPTER FIVE

WHEN TO START PREPARING FOR LABOR AND DELIVERY

When should you start preparing for the big day? Honestly, there's no exact timeline. But the earlier you start thinking about it, the less you'll feel overwhelmed as the date approaches.

Preparing for Labor: It's All About Being Ready (and Flexible)

- Childbirth Classes: These classes are amazing because they give you the tools and confidence to understand what's happening to your body.

- Packing Your Hospital Bag: Pack your bag at least a month before your due date. Bring comfortable clothes, wipes, toiletries, snacks (for you), and anything that'll make you feel comfortable like your pregnancy pillow for example. I've seen a lot of women bring their robe and slippers to the delivery room so do no feel embarrassed because whether or not you like to be the center of attention this experience will be about you and you need to embrace it.

- Creating a Birth Plan: Your birth plan is like a wish list, not a script. Things might not go as planned, and that's ok. But it helps to be prepared and have your preferences noted.

Labor Can Be Unpredictable

Labor might go smoothly, or it might throw you a few curveballs.
Whatever happens, trust that your body knows what to do. Lean on your support system—partner, family, friends, or healthcare team—and know that it's okay to ask for help when you need it.

Tips: There are a few holistic remedies that are know to make labor easier.
Okra water, raspberry tea, walking and pregnancy yoga.
Feel free to inform yourself and choose a method that works for you.

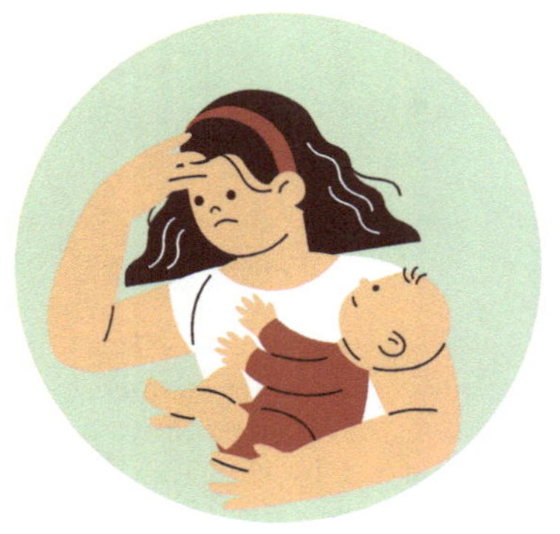

CHAPTER SIX

POSTPARTUM & TAKING CARE OF BABY

You've made it through pregnancy and childbirth—and now comes the recovery and the care of your newborn. It's a time filled with new challenges, but also immense joy.

Navigating Postpartum Recovery

I know, you read this throughout the whole book but I will repeat myself again: you need to take care of yourself. Your body was used as a vessel to bring life on earth and it will need time to heal. It's okay to rest, to ask for help, and to lean into the support of those around you. You're not expected to do everything perfectly and especially alone.

Caring for Baby: One Step at a Time

Taking care of your newborn is a learning process. You'll get into a rhythm with feeding, changing, and soothing your little one. There is no need to be anxious about a good time to feed because your baby will let you know. Trust your instincts—they'll guide you. Most women experience a natural protective mechanism after birth which allows them to nurture a lot more easily.

You are enough mama !

As you step into motherhood, remember that you don't need to be perfect. You just need to be you. And you are more than enough. It's okay to feel overwhelmed, to question your decisions, or to need help. What matters most is the bond you're building with your baby—and that's what will carry you through.
Take a deep breath. Trust the process. And remember that you are loved, you are capable, and you've got this.

AFFIRMATION CARDS

I trust my body to
know what to do.

I welcome my
changing body with
gratitude.

I make the best
decisions for me and
my baby.

One day/moment at
a time.

AFFIRMATION CARDS

I find the positives in each day of my pregnancy.

My baby feels safe and peaceful in my womb.

I will create my own positive birth experience.

I am capable of amazing things.

notes

DATE   /   /

notes

DATE   /   /

notes

DATE   /   /

THANK
You

Sincerely,

Noémi Woynin

9 798302 974938